# LAST KNOWN CONTACT

## The Untold Story of
## Luigi Mangione

Author

**Anonymous**

ISBN: 9781965560754

# Dedication

*This book is dedicated to those who strive to understand the complexities of humanity and to those who seek justice and truth in a world often blurred by systems and narratives.*

# Acknowledgments

I would like to express my deepest gratitude to the individuals who shared their perspectives, stories, and memories of Luigi Mangione. Your insights and reflections have shaped this narrative in profound ways. To the journalists, thank you for your support and thinkers who pursue truth amidst the chaos; thank you for your tireless efforts. And to those who navigate the complexities of life with empathy and courage, this work is for you.

# Table of Contents

# Introduction

The Beginning of the Mystery The day Luigi Mangione's name became synonymous with scandal was the day my life was divided into two parts: before and after. To the world, Luigi was infamous, linked to the death of UnitedHealthcare CEO Brian Thompson in a case that captivated global attention. But to me, Luigi was a friend—someone I had shared adventures with during my travels in Southeast Asia, someone I laughed and debated with. Reconciling the Luigi, I knew with the one portrayed in the headlines felt impossible, as if two entirely different individuals were being forced into the same frame.

It began on an ordinary night at 2 a.m. in Da Nang, Vietnam. I had been living there for months, enjoying a peaceful routine. My days started with the sound of waves crashing, a refreshing morning swim, and a mango-pineapple smoothie at my favorite juice bar. I'd spend hours in a local coffee shop, working on freelance marketing projects, feeling grounded in my routine.

That night, during a call with my best friend about fantasy football, a news alert flashed on my phone. At first, it didn't register. Then, I saw the photo. Luigi's photo. My chest tightened. "Bro," I whispered, my voice trembling, "I think I know him. I think I know Luigi."

My friend dismissed it as a coincidence, but I couldn't shake the feeling. I opened Instagram to confirm. The sinking realization became undeniable: the man in the CNN photo was Luigi. "This is Luigi," I said urgently. "Me and Sabastian met him in Bangkok. I can't believe this shit."

Within hours, my social media exploded. Journalists flooded my inbox, hungry for any insight about Luigi. Andre Tinko from CBS News, Victoria Cox from Inside Edition, and Nicholas Bogel-

Burroughs from The New York Times all reached out. My peaceful existence in Da Nang shattered, replaced by a whirlwind of memories, questions, and doubts.

Our paths had first crossed in Bangkok, Thailand, in March 2024. It was my first trip to Asia, and I was eager to explore. I had left the U.S. to travel the continent, taking on freelance work and vlogging for my channel, my YouTube channel. My guide was Sabastian, a professional soccer player and Thailand resident for over three years. One evening, Sabastian suggested we visit Soi Cowboy, a street famed for its neon-lit bars.

We ended up at Stumble Inn Cowboy, sitting on the balcony, sipping beers and watching the street's bustling energy. That's when Luigi walked in alone and took a seat at a table near ours. Sabastian noticed his American accent and struck up a conversation. Luigi smiled and joined us, introducing himself.

From that first interaction, Luigi stood out. He was confident yet restless, magnetic yet enigmatic. He laughed at my Mario-inspired joke about his name and engaged us in deeper conversations as the night wore on. His openness about his real name in hindsight, surprising given his later reputation for using aliases suggested he trusted us.

Our initial conversations covered typical topics: travel, hometowns, and aspirations. But Luigi's sharp insights and eclectic interests soon emerged. We debated politics and societal systems, with Luigi passionately criticizing corporate greed and systemic corruption. His insights were profound, backed by books he'd read and experiences he'd lived. Even Sabastian, often quick to challenge others, found himself agreeing with Luigi's logic.

That night, under the glow of Bangkok's nightlife scene. Luigi's charm and intellect made an unforgettable impression. Yet, none of us could have imagined the scandal that would later engulf his name.

The times following that first meeting were a whirlwind of exploration. Luigi became a regular part of our group, joining us on various adventures throughout Thailand. We visited temples and immersed ourselves in the cultural of Thailand. Luigi's enthusiasm for history and architecture was evident in every conversation. He was curiosity and had high energy; encouraging all of us to see the world through different perspectives.

As the months passed, our group eventually went our separate ways. Luigi returned to the U.S. while I continued my travels across Asia. We stayed in touch through social media, exchanging messages and photos.

Then came the news. The Luigi I knew, the friend I meet in Bangkok was now at the center of a global scandal.

# Chapter 1

# Meeting Luigi

I first met Luigi Mangione in March 2024 in Bangkok at a bar called Stumble Inn Cowboy, nestled in the heart of the infamous Soi Cowboy Road. The neon-lit strip, buzzing with energy, was a sensory overload of flashing lights, booming music, and travelers and locals from all over the world. As someone new to both Bangkok and Asia, I was captivated by the chaos and vibrancy of it all.

I had recently left the United States to explore Southeast Asia, picking up freelance technical marketing projects to fund my travels. My YouTube channel, is an attempt to document my experiences and share the vibrancy of life on the road. That night, my GoPro was strapped to my chest, ready to capture whatever the night had in store. My guide to Bangkok's streets was my friend Sabastian, a professional soccer player who had lived in Thailand for over three years. When he suggested, we visit Soi Cowboy, a street famed for its LED-lit bars and unfiltered nightlife. I said, "Yes, let's do it." Little did I know that I would meet Luigi that night!

We eventually wandered into Stumble Inn Cowboy, a bar with an inviting balcony overlooking the lively street. As we drank our beers and watched the crowds below, a man walked in and immediately caught my attention—not because of his appearance, but because of his presence. Luigi had effortless confidence about him, paired with a subtle restlessness that made it seem like he was always ready to move, to pivot, to adapt.

Luigi sat at a table near us alone and ordered a beer. Sabastian, sitting closest to him, picked up on his American accent immediately. "Where are you from? I know you're American," Sabastian said, his tone friendly and welcoming. Luigi smiled and turned toward us; his expression relaxed yet watchful. After a brief exchange, we invited him to join our table, and he accepted without hesitation.

He introduced himself simply as Luigi. The name struck me immediately, and I couldn't resist making a joke. "You probably hear this a lot," I said, grinning, "but you're the only Luigi I've ever met. I had to do it." He laughed, the sound breaking any lingering tension, and from that moment on, the conversation flowed effortlessly.

At the time, I didn't think much about the simplicity of his introduction. It was only later, after his arrest, that I learned how frequently Luigi used fake IDs and aliases during his travels. In hindsight, it became clear that our connection that night was genuine enough for him to use his real name an unusual act for someone as guarded as Luigi.

Our initial conversation was light and filled with the typical traveler questions: "Where are you from?" "What brought you to Bangkok?" "What do you do for a living?" Sabastian and I are both Texas boys, and Luigi mentioned that he was in the AI tech space and from Texas. I myself and in the AI space while Sabastian and am an athlete by profession. Sabastian, a massive Pokémon fan, shifted the topic to vintage Gameboys when Luigi noticed one on the table. Luigi's excitement about the Gameboy led to a nostalgic conversation about childhood gaming, evolving into broader discussions about Halo, Diablo, and our favorite childhood games.

As the beers flowed, our conversations grew more meaningful. We debated politics, personal aspirations, and the broader frustrations of navigating a world that often felt rigged. Luigi's thoughts on societal systems came through early on. He expressed frustration with systems like healthcare, politics, and the economy, which he saw as benefiting the few while keeping the majority in line. At the time, his words felt like the musings of a frustrated traveler, but in retrospect, they carried deeper insight.

A good bar story always has a hint of scandal a mix of truth and intrigue that keeps you questioning what's real and what's embellished. With Luigi, there was always that edge, a sense that there was more beneath the surface of his words. He wasn't just offering wild theories; he explained his points with references and examples, breaking things down in a way that made connections clear. His critiques of corporate greed, for instance, felt grounded in universal truths, resonating with the frustrations of many Americans.

He backed his claims with data and examples, often referencing books, documentaries, or historical events. He described the healthcare system, the banking industry, and political lobbying with a confidence that came from deep understanding, not just surface-level outrage. He often pointed out that the system worked exactly as designed to benefit the few at the expense of the many.

There was a sharpness to his insights that night, the kind of intelligence that made you sit up and pay attention. Luigi wasn't some random guy at the bar rambling after a few drinks he was deliberate, articulate, and often unsettlingly accurate. Even Sabastian, who was usually quick to debate, found himself agreeing more often than not. Luigi's arguments weren't just compelling; they were backed by logic and a breadth of knowledge that made them hard to dismiss.

Looking back, it was both fascinating and a little unnerving. It wasn't just what he said, but how he said it confidently, unapologetically, like he had already weighed every possible counterargument and found them lacking. He wasn't naive or ignorant. If anything, he seemed to know too much, and for a moment that night, sitting under the neon glow of Soi Cowboy, it felt like we were seeing the world through his eyes.

Luigi had a knack for captivating his audience, and that night was no exception. We played a drinking game, betting on which passersby would enter the ladyboy bars versus the regular ones. Luigi, with an uncanny ability to read people's body language, won nearly every round. With a smirk on his face, he mentioned that you can recognize it by whether they hesitate or not. For a while, his laughter was infectious, and the weight of his cynicism seemed to lift.

As the night wore on and the bar began to empty, Luigi started sharing pieces of his past. He grew up in Baltimore, Maryland, the middle child in a family that emphasized success and appearances. His father, a real estate developer, had instilled a relentless drive for achievement in his children. Luigi, however, felt like he didn't fit the mold. He described his time at an all-boys private school as both a privilege and a prison.

I joked about his background, saying, *"Oh, so you're rich rich,"* attempting to lighten the mood and acknowledging his wealth because, coming from a public-school background, I understood that private schools like his cost around $30k a year. He laughed but didn't deny it. He reflected on how that environment taught him to play the game but left him feeling like an outsider. While many people wanted things like a big mansion or a fancy car, he didn't.

I joked with him again, saying, *"It's easy to be humble when you're rich and to want less when you already have more."* He chuckled, and I shared how I came from humble beginnings and saw my family rise financially during my teenage years. I admitted that I wasn't like him in that regard.

I told him, *"I've been working illegally since I was 15. I've had a job ever since—sometimes two jobs—while going to college. Even now, I've been grinding nonstop. It's safe to say it's not fun. And boy, would I have loved to know that my bloodline was secured, with no worries throughout life."*

One moment from that night stayed with me. As we sat under the neon glow of Soi Cowboy, Luigi turned to me and shared a thought about the futility of trying to win in a rigged game. It was a sentiment that struck a chord, resonating in a way I didn't fully understand at the time.

Luigi's demeanor that night was a fascinating blend of charm and guardedness. He had a way of opening up just enough to draw you in but never so much that you felt you truly knew him. His insights were sharp, often backed by books he had read or experiences he had lived. Despite his cynicism, there was a clear passion for understanding the world and finding solutions to its problems.

That night marked the beginning of a friendship that would later take on an entirely different significance. At the time, it was just a night of good conversation, shared beers, and lighthearted fun in the vibrant chaos of Bangkok. Looking back, it feels like the prelude to a story I never saw coming.

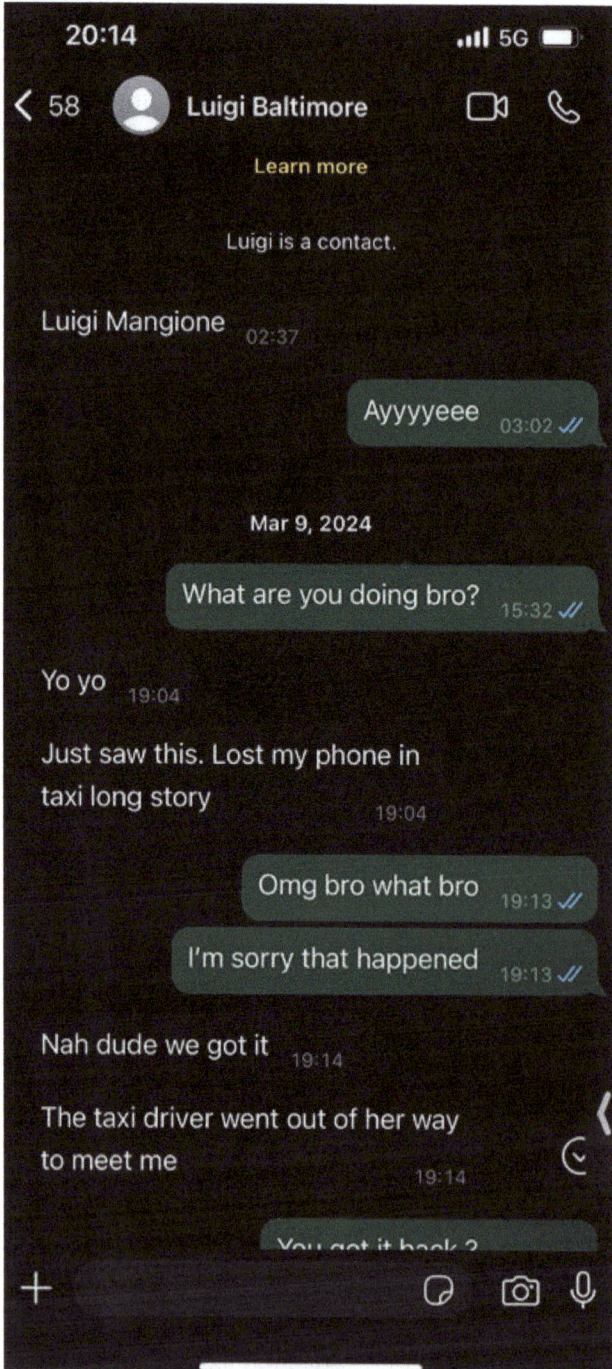

# Chapter 2

# Adventures in Bangkok

In 2024, Bangkok's nightlife became our playground, and Luigi thrived in its chaos. From dive bars to rooftop lounges, he navigated the city with a magnetic energy that drew people in. He had a way of making even the most mundane nights feel like an adventure.

One night stands out vividly. We were at a smoky bar, surrounded by a mix of ex-pats and locals, when Luigi got into a heated argument with a group of ladyboys. Although I was not there for the fight and left earlier, I found it funny. He told me what began as a playful exchange quickly escalated into a full-blown brawl. Drinks spilled, voices rose, and chaos erupted. By the end of it, Luigi had scratches all over his body and a couple of bruises.

That memory came rushing back another night when Luigi called me after I'd gone home early. His voice was a mix of disbelief and amusement as he launched into what had unfolded after I left. He and a few guys he'd just met decided to check out one of the infamous sex bars. They all went in together, had about two beers each, and when the bill came, it totaled a jaw-dropping 50,000 baht or around $1,500 USD. I was stunned and immediately asked how well he knew these guys, suggesting that maybe one of them had ordered a little something on the side to inflate the tab.

He explained that they were all there just drinking, and he believed someone had tried to scam them, assuming they were too drunk to notice. That, as it turned out, was just the beginning. When they started questioning the bill, things escalated quickly, and the group found themselves surrounded and attacked by ladyboys from all sides.

By the time he got to that part, I was practically doubled over with laughter, tears streaming down my face at the sheer absurdity of it all.

He tried to keep his composure, but even he couldn't help laughing as he recounted the chaos. What struck me about the whole ordeal was how unabashedly he told the story. Most people would have buried a moment like that, embarrassed or ashamed. But Luigi wore it like a badge of honor, scratches and all. Later that night, he sent me a photo of the aftermath a series of red scratches from the scuffle, proof of the wild night that had unfolded.

It wasn't just funny; it was oddly disarming. His openness and humor about the whole thing had a way of putting people at ease, myself included. It made me feel comfortable enough to share my own stories, including deeper issues I usually kept buried family struggles, personal doubts, and, yes, my share of crazy nights. That was the kind of person Luigi was. He could take a ridiculous, over-the-top moment and turn it into a story you'd never forget. In doing so, he made it easier for those around him to be vulnerable, real, and unfiltered in return. When you hear stories like this, it's natural to share epic nights and experiences you've had as well. It's easy to let your guard down because he speaks genuinely. To be fair, more often than not, I find that some of the smartest people I know many friends making well beyond six figures in engineering and tech; tend to party hard every once in a while; the yin to their intelligent yang.

Despite his wild side, Luigi had a thoughtful complexity that surfaced in quieter moments. On nights when the city seemed to slow down, he would sit after eating, overlooking the city while sharing his thoughts on life. He often referenced the Unabomber's critiques of societal greed and technological overreach, admiring the unfiltered commentary on how modern systems perpetuate inequality and corruption. For Luigi, these were truths he believed shaped the broken world we lived in.

Music became another way for him to process and reflect. His playlists spanned everything from classic rock to obscure indie tracks, and he had a knack for picking songs that fit the mood perfectly. Even his humor carried an edge of irreverence. Luigi wore a wristband labeled "Cum Boy," I asked him why you got that one, he was like it was a joke. Then I showed him my mind because I bought the same style of different works that read "Mr. Fuck" just another gag tourists picked up as a lighthearted joke. For both of us, these wristbands were a humorous not to be taken seriously.

His social media posts mirrored this duality. They captured his ability to find peace in chaos and beauty in disorder, offering rare glimpses into the mind of someone who existed effortlessly at the crossroads of wild abandon and quiet reflection.

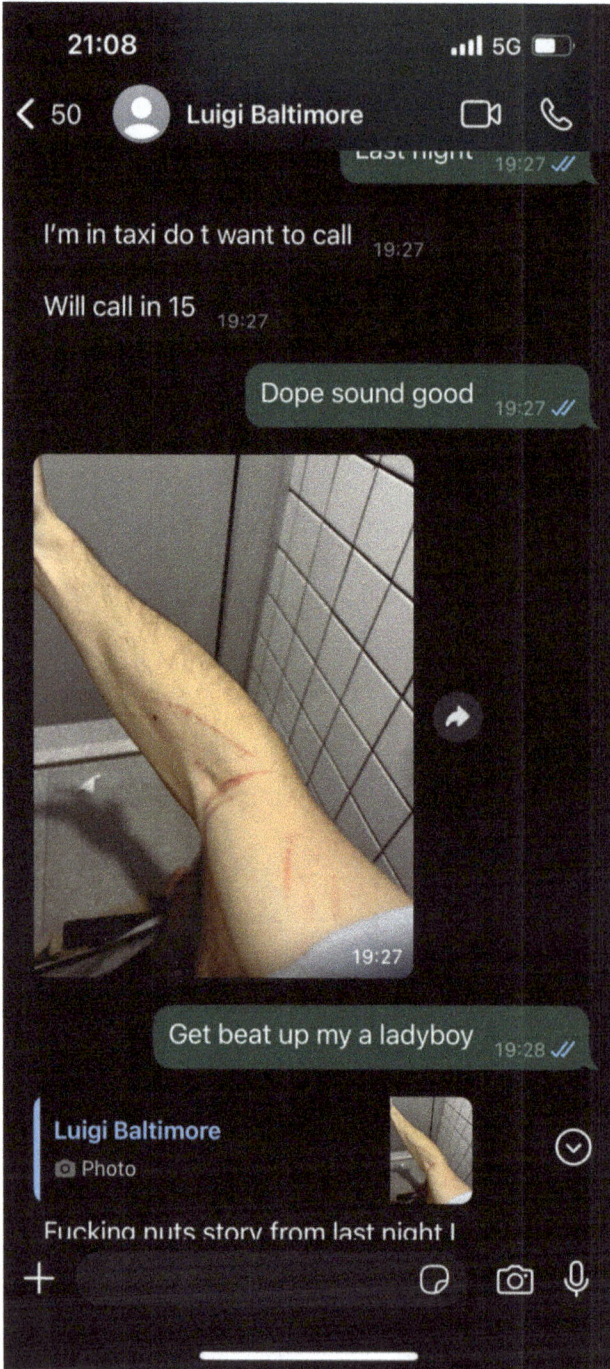

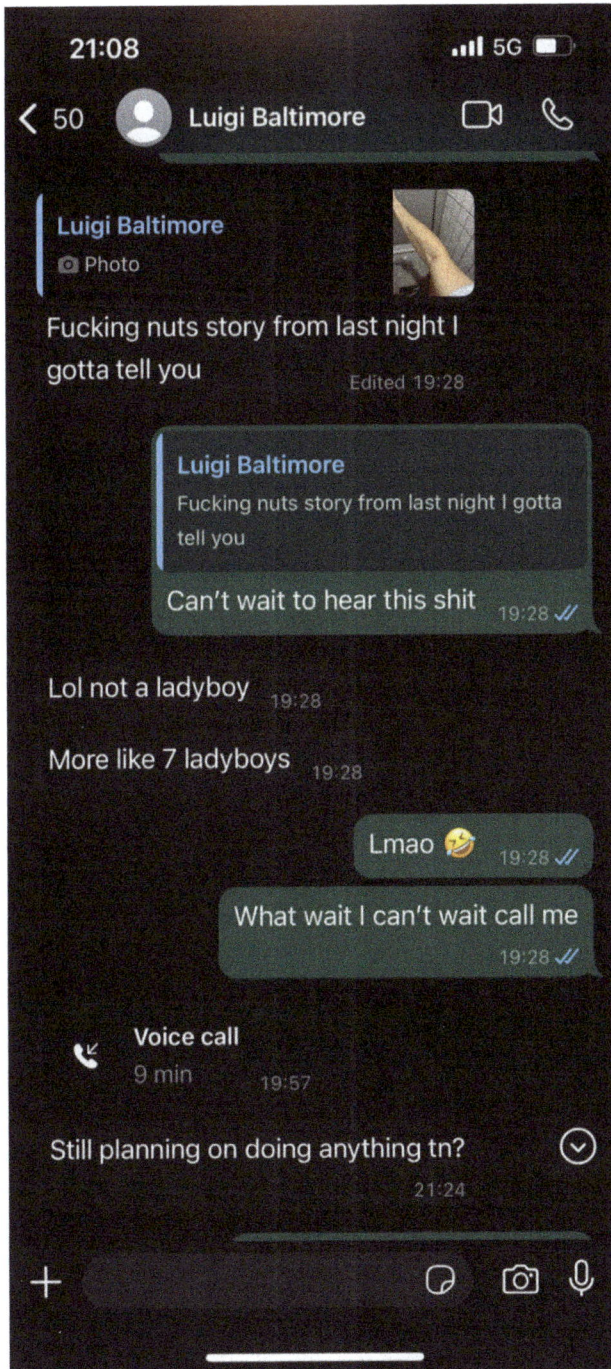

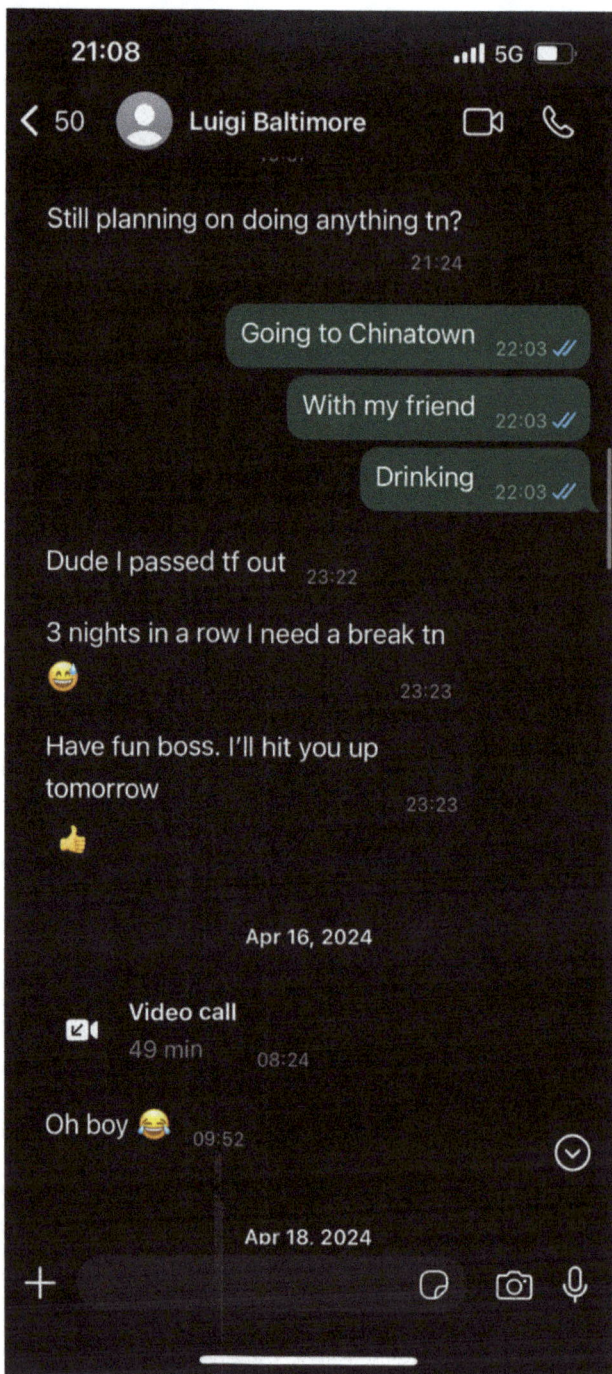

21:08 　　　　　　　📶 5G 🔋

< 50 　👤 **Luigi Baltimore** 　　📹 📞

Still planning on doing anything tn?
21:24

Going to Chinatown 22:03 ✓✓

With my friend 22:03 ✓✓

Drinking 22:03 ✓✓

Dude I passed tf out 23:22

3 nights in a row I need a break tn
😅 　　　　　　　23:23

Have fun boss. I'll hit you up
tomorrow
23:23
👍

Apr 16, 2024

📹 **Video call**
49 min 　08:24

Oh boy 😂 09:52 　　　　　　⌄

Apr 18, 2024

\+ 　　　　　　　🗨 📷 🎤

# Chapter 3
# Searching for Meaning

Beneath the chaos and revelry of Bangkok's nightlife, Luigi was a man deeply in search of meaning. His restless energy often disguised an introspective side that emerged only in quieter moments. He had a voracious appetite for books, gravitating toward those that challenged societal norms. One of the most compelling conversations I had with Luigi revolved around two books that deeply shaped his worldview: *Confessions of an Economic Hitman* by John Perkins and *The Unabomber Manifesto* by Ted Kaczynski. Luigi, ever the intellectual, drew parallels between the predatory tactics described in Perkins' book and the warnings Kaczynski issued about unchecked technological advancement.

Rather than focusing on resource extraction, Luigi pointed to the rise of automation and artificial intelligence as a modern example of Kaczynski's predictions. Kaczynski had warned of a world where technology would become so pervasive that it would strip humanity of its autonomy, forcing people to conform to systems designed to serve the technology itself rather than the individuals it was meant to help. Luigi saw this playing out in industries like transportation, manufacturing, and customer service, where automation has replaced countless jobs. He highlighted how self-driving cars, AI-powered customer support systems, and fully automated factories are reshaping the labor market.

Luigi's concern wasn't just about job displacement; it was about the erosion of purpose and identity for those affected. He spoke about the psychological toll this shift takes on people, particularly those whose roles become obsolete. Workers aren't just losing jobs; they're losing their sense of contribution and value in a society increasingly driven by efficiency over humanity.

For Luigi, the parallels to Kaczynski's warnings were stark. Kaczynski feared that once society became overly reliant on technology, it would create systems so complex and interdependent that individuals would have no choice but to adapt to them or be left behind. Luigi believed we were already seeing this in action. As automation and AI become more ingrained in daily life, people are forced to accept changes they can't control; whether it's navigating an automated customer service system or adapting to new, tech-driven roles in the workplace.

The example Luigi found most chilling was the growing role of AI in decision-making processes, from hiring practices to judicial rulings. These systems, he argued, these systems were unregulated and riddled with biases inherited from their creators. Yet, society increasingly relies on them, surrendering critical decisions to algorithms that prioritize efficiency over ethics. This, Luigi believed, was the ultimate realization of Kaczynski's fears: a world where technology not only replaces human labor but also governs human behavior.

Reflecting on our conversation, I couldn't help but see the truth from Luigi's perspective. The integration of AI and automation has undoubtedly brought convenience and progress, but it has also raised questions about the human cost. How much autonomy are we willing to sacrifice in the name of efficiency? And what happens to those who are left behind in this relentless march toward technological dominance?

Luigi frequently reflected on the themes from these books, dissecting their critiques of greed, power structures, and the exploitation of the masses. He would describe them as exposing the unsettling truth that the world was engineered to benefit the few at the expense of the many. These weren't just abstract ideas to him; his words carried a bitterness that felt deeply personal as if he had spent years grappling with these realizations and the disillusionment they brought.

One topic that came up repeatedly in our conversations was healthcare. It was a subject that seemed to ignite a unique fury in Luigi, perhaps because it felt so universally broken and deeply unfair. The disparity between Thailand's affordable care and the exorbitant costs in the U.S. became glaringly obvious during our time in Bangkok.

One incident particularly enraged him: when our friend Sabastian injured his knee and received treatment for just $150. The X-ray scans cost only $15, and the remaining $135 covered the actual surgery. Luigi was visibly upset as he gestured toward Sabastian's bandaged leg, pointing out how this was what healthcare was supposed to look like—helping people, not bankrupting them. He mentioned how an X-ray alone would cost significantly more in the U.S., let alone the cost of surgery.

The subject hit close to home for all of us. Luigi often recounted his own struggle with a costly back surgery that hadn't even resolved his pain. I shared my own experience of tearing my Achilles the year before, explaining how, even with company insurance, my deductible was an astronomical $12,000, but surgery its well totaled over 80k without rehab. Luigi's frustration boiled over as he questioned how anyone could justify such a system.

He often expressed his frustration, saying that capitalism was crushing Americans. With a mix of anger and disbelief, he pointed out how pharmaceutical companies charged anywhere from $100 to $1,000 for pills that cost mere pennies to produce. He questioned how such a system could be called healthcare, emphasizing the irony of being the richest nation while failing to provide proper care for its people.

When I replied with a simple *"Greed,"* it felt like the only answer that could encapsulate the systemic rot we were talking about. Luigi nodded, his expression grim, as though the conversation merely confirmed what he already believed: the system was irredeemably corrupt.

He mentioned how all insurance companies participate in these practices and expressed his frustration at how the American healthcare system has been overtaken by such greed. *"It's disrespectful to the American people,"* He mentioned Brian Thompson and his leadership at United Healthcare, noting the massive profit influx the company has seen since he took over. At the same time, Luigi pointed out, denials for claims have seemingly increased, raising questions about the cost of those profits and who ultimately bears the burden.

What struck me most was how personal Luigi made these discussions. He wasn't just reciting facts or statistics; he empathized on a deeply human level. Despite his upbringing private boarding school and an affluent family background he spoke with genuine care and passion for the struggles of everyday Americans. His ability to connect across class lines was rare and deeply resonant.

Luigi's love for tattoos was another reflection of his search for identity and meaning. During our wanderings through Bangkok's streets, we often stopped to admire tattoo shops, looking at some different designs that we could potentially get. He talked about wanting something we could never really settle on a design to get.

Music offered yet another outlet for his introspection. Luigi's playlists were eclectic, ranging from classic rock to obscure indie and experimental genres.

Luigi mentioned how he love volcanos; and how he lived in Hawaii and how being there was so peaceful. He showed me pictures of roads being destroyed from a volcano. I mentioned the power of volcanos and the healing waters that comes from it due to hot water springs. These volcanic hot water springs contains sulfur and magnesium both of which are good for the body and for healing. Luigi was not aware of that component and I was happy to share some of the knowledge I am learned about it. I explained the natural healing methods of geothermal springs and the power of traditional medicine with an individual named Dr Sebi; who managed to cure diseases such as diabetes HIV and other major illnesses. Luigi was not aware of these finds and listened. I told him Dr. Sebi won a court case in New York Supreme court again Big Pharma by proving that these illnesses could be cured by eliminating mucus from the body and having and alkaline diet. Though Dr. Sebi did not have a doctoral degree to practice medicine he was still able to cure many individually with his methods. I told him at one point Left Eye of TLC and Michael Jackson where some of his clients although not a lot of media surrounds his time with those. I explained how during his trial he brought over 20 witnesses including licensed use doctors that were baffled that and uneducated "doctor" could have cured these illnesses without formal training. If convicted of practicing false medicine Dr. Sebi was facing the rest of his life in jail but the witnesses help prove his innocence. After winning the trial Dr. Sebi mentioned in his own words that when a break through happens in medical field he expected all the doctors and pharmaceutical companies to get behind his cause as the new medical standard to cure diseases. Dr Sebi quickly realized that the opposite happened not only did the medical community not accept him but they also shunned him. All of this information was new to Luigi and he was intrigued to understand more about it even looking up the case on his phone right away. In closing out discussion I mentioned how he died under mysterious circumstances in Mexico. I told Luigi no one ever knows what actually happened but this would not be the first-time people die under stranger conditions when they have something that could jeopardize the billions of dollars the medical industry makes. People who try to do right by society are often punished and die weird and unusual deaths.

Luigi's ability to navigate between chaos and introspection was what made him so compelling. One moment, he'd be recounting a wild story from a Bangkok bar, laughing about the absurdity of a scuffle with ladyboys over a padded tab; the next, he'd be dissecting the failures of the healthcare system who saw the wheels of its injustice.

Of all the topics Luigi delved into, healthcare resonated with him the most because it offended him on a deeply personal level. It wasn't just an abstract critique of a broken system; it was a wound he carried with him every day with injuries. His own experience with an expensive back surgery that failed to fully heal his pain left him upset with the way he was treated. He felt betrayed by a system that seemed to prioritize profits over people's well-being. Every conversation about healthcare brought a sharp edge to his voice, as though the injustice of it all struck at the core of his values. For Luigi, the exploitation embedded in the industry wasn't just another example of corporate greed it was a violation of what he believed should be the most basic human right: the ability to receive care without being financially destroyed in the process.

Luigi and I never spoke about committing a crime, but I remember one conversation where I told him. There's nothing to be done. It's too late. We live in a world ruled by money, taxes, and systems that don't truly serve us. Unfortunately, it is our modern reality we live in. I told him how we're all living in a circus, distracted by screens, TV shows, sports, and endless streams of digital content. These distractions keep us from focusing on the real issues, the ones that affect our lives in profound ways, like healthcare and government accountability.

Luigi agreed, adding that if people spent less time consumed by digital media and more time paying attention to what their governments were doing, or what they were allowing to happen, things might change. He pointed out how the constant consumption of entertainment leaves us blind to the bigger picture. He mentioned that they've engineered it that way, and if they keep people entertained and distracted, then they will never question the system. It was sobering to hear, but it's true. We are washed up in a system drowning in the forever cycle to consume; whether that's media or treatments to keep bringing in medical bill checks.

Luigi's had a lot to say when it came on his perspective on healthcare. He was appalled by the stark contrast between the U.S. system and those in countries often labeled as "third world." He questioned how the country could claim to be the best when healthcare costs were a hundred times higher than in other nations, despite the expectation of being number one. He shared examples of how treatments in Southeast Asia could cost a fraction of what they do in America sometimes just 1% of the price. And despite the lower costs, the care was often better without the bureaucracy and gatekeeping of insurance companies. Pharmacies were accessible, medications were affordable, and people weren't burdened by the fear of financial ruin for seeking basic medical help.

It was mind-blowing to think about. In countries with far fewer resources, healthcare was structured to prioritize accessibility and affordability for all people. Meanwhile, in the wealthiest nation on Earth, the system seemed designed to prioritize profit over people. Luigi's frustration mirrored my own, and our conversation left me questioning how much longer we could sustain such a broken model. It was one of those moments where you realize just how far we've strayed from the ideals we claim to uphold, and it made me wonder: What would it take for us to wake up and demand better?

## Religious Reflections and Corruption

We often delved into the topic of religion, and as always, our conversations were both deep and thought-provoking. Luigi admitted that he wasn't particularly religious. He admitted that he didn't really believe in anything. In response, I shared my perspective, explaining that for me, religion came down to sticking with the "guy that got me to the party." I told him how Sabastian faith and mine had been a guiding force, helping me navigate life's challenges. "There's been too many coincidences," I said, "even in science, for me to ignore. Somebody had to put this plan together. The way everything connects how one plant can heal an ailment caused by another in the same region of the world, or how there's always a balance; it's too perfect to be random."

Luigi listened intently, not arguing but instead sharing his frustrations. He mentioned that he didn't believe the great Creator existed because he saw too much wrong in the world to believe in anything. The conversation shifted to the question of who, if anyone, rules the earth.

I told him, *"To be honest, I don't think God rules the earth. I think the other guy does. This is an evil game, and evil lurks at the top."* In contrast, I pointed out that many of the laws in modern societies are rooted in the Ten Commandments. I explained that not everything in the Bible should be taken literally. Instead, much of it can be interpreted as analogies, hidden messages, principles of science, and universal truths embedded in its stories.

I told him that by not reading it even if you're not religious and lean more toward spirituality you rob yourself of ancient knowledge.

To my surprise, Luigi agreed. The powers that be whatever you want to call them they're insidious. It's like they've designed everything to benefit themselves, no matter the cost. We joked about how they were like the Sith from *Star Wars*, wielding immense power in secret and ensuring that wrongdoing thrived unchecked. Yet, even in our cynicism, we both agreed on one universal truth: no matter what religion someone follows or even if they follow none at all wrong is wrong. The systems in place like healthcare, the suffering they perpetuate, and the greed they foster are undeniable. Unfortunately, we also recognized that so much of the wrong in the world is allowed to pass without challenge, and that realization lingered long after the conversation ended.

As Luigi and I spoke, our discussion delved into the nature of power and how knowledge can be wielded for both good and evil. I explained that knowledge itself isn't inherently bad it's like fire. In the right hands, it can provide warmth and light; in the wrong hands, it can burn and destroy.

We touched on the topic of Freemasonry, agreeing that it's not necessarily the Freemasons themselves who are evil, but rather how their knowledge is applied, that determines the outcome, especially given the existence of many different factions. Luigi emphasized that power in general leads to corruption pointing out how evil tends to thrive in the highest positions of authority.

We reflected on corruption as a Hydra cut off one head and two more grow in its place. The system is a machine, and removing one corrupt individual won't stop it; the machine itself perpetuates the cycle. I told Luigi that eliminating corruption would require a complete dismantling of the system of corrupted individuals, akin to snapping one's fingers with the power of Thanos. Even then, I wasn't sure it would be enough. "The next generation will just inherit power," I said. "And power inevitably corrupts." Luigi agreed, noting how even those with good intentions often lose their way over time. We joked, half-seriously, that it would take unshakable integrity and savior-like figures immune to bribery or greed to bring true change. In the end, we acknowledged the uncomfortable truth: the cycle continues, and the challenge of stopping it feels unachievable.

## Sports, Manipulation, and Luigi's Morality

Even when discussing sports, Luigi and I couldn't avoid diving into its underlying power dynamics. We liked to think sports were one of the last pure forms of competition, but even there, manipulation seemed inevitable. College football, we agreed, might be the last bastion of purity a space where stakes feel genuine and untainted by corporate greed.

One memorable discussion revolved around the Tyson fight versus Jake Paul. Luigi's perspective was typically blunt; he believed that if Tyson was even half of his usual self in the first few rounds, the fight would be over. However, he also noted that there was no way Vegas would allow itself to lose billions on this fight.

Breaking it down, Luigi explained how betting odds often favor the house Vegas rarely loses. He concluded that the smart bet was on Jake, believing that outcomes usually serve the system, not the sport. As much as I wanted to argue, I couldn't; Luigi's reasoning was as convincing as ever.

We both recognized that Vegas is not in the business of losing billions. It's not built for people to win consistently if they did, Vegas simply wouldn't exist.

Luigi's understanding of manipulation wasn't limited to sports. He saw these patterns everywhere from politics to entertainment and believed they reflected deeper truths about human nature and society's structures. This perspective, while often cynical, underscored his enduring search for morality in an immoral world. It wasn't just about identifying what was wrong; it was about finding the strength to live authentically despite it.

Through all his critiques and frustrations, Luigi remained driven by a restless hope a belief that even in a rigged system, moments of meaning and connection could still be found. It was this hope, tempered by his sharp intellect and raw honesty, that made him unforgettable.

## Luigi's Vision for the Future

I often think of the future and how these could have been different and he echoed those thoughts as well. He imagined a world where systems worked for people rather than against them. He believed in small actions that could ripple outward moments of kindness, grassroots movements, and personal integrity. He once mentioned that you don't have to change everything. Making a single change for someone could be a good starting point. It was a philosophy he carried in the way he treated people with curiosity, empathy, and a willingness to listen.

In many ways, Luigi's vision was both idealistic and grounded. He knew the world wouldn't change overnight, but he believed in the power of persistence. Whether through meaningful conversations, music, or simply sharing a laugh, he found ways to create moments that mattered.

# Chapter 4

# Fading Connections

As our time together wound down, Luigi began to pull away. He talked less about his family and friends back home and more about the freedom of anonymity. He had missed a close friend's wedding, a decision he brushed off but one that clearly weighed on him. It was as though he was gradually detaching himself from the ties that had once grounded him, seeking peaceful life away from American modern society.

Luigi often spoke with admiration about Japan, and one particular conversation about his plans to visit there stands out vividly in my memory. I had mentioned to him that I'd never been to Japan but would love to go someday, and his face lit up as he began describing it. His enthusiasm was obvious as he told me I would love it. He painted a picture of the streets illuminated by vibrant LED lights, reminiscent of the ones we had seen on Soi Cowboy in Thailand but taken to a whole new level. Moreover, he mentioned that it's kind of like walking in a futuristic movie set. The way he spoke, it was clear that Japan's blend of tradition and modernity fascinated him.

But then the conversation took a deeper turn. Luigi started talking about how Japan's technological advancements had inadvertently created societal challenges with the declining birth rate. He attributed this issue to a combination of factors, many of which were tied to technology. Luigi believed that the overstimulation provided by tech endless streams of entertainment, social media, and virtual interactions was replacing genuine human connections. He pointed out that people are more stimulated by their phones than by real human interaction, pointing out that technology is starting to outweigh biology.

Luigi also spoke about the anxiety fueled by a hyperconnected world, where people were constantly comparing themselves to curated versions of others' lives online. He saw Japan as a case study for the unintended consequences of progress, where innovation had outpaced the ability to address its societal impacts. To him, it was a cautionary tale about the double-edged sword of technological advancements. As much as Luigi admired Japan's cutting-edge tech and cultural vibrancy, he couldn't help but reflect on the broader implications of a society increasingly mediated by screens rather than human touch.

He once told me that sometimes it's easier to disappear. It wasn't just his friends and family he ghosted; he was leaving behind his past and wanted to find himself.

Luigi mentioned during one of our late-night conversations that his disconnect from his family had grown since his time in Hawaii. He shared images of volcanoes with me and destructive power of roads that had melted away from lava and vocalic eruption. I believe he had

We also delved into Luigi's fascination with conspiracy theories during this phase. He often talked about how every theory, no matter how wild, contained "bits of the truth." He believed that to get to the heart of the matter, you need to follow the money, as that's where the real story is. One night, he referenced a line from *Rush Hour*, joking that in every scandal or misdeed, there's a rich figure benefiting from the chaos.

He expanded on this with examples of modern industries, including the EV movement and its ties to cobalt mining in nations like the Democratic Republic of Congo. Luigi's disdain for exploitation and systemic greed became a recurring theme in our talks. He also brought up the ideas explored in *Confessions of an Economic Hit Man*, particularly how countries with valuable resources like those powering the technological advancements of our generation are often exploited.

He mentioned that some tech companies don't act in good faith. They would rather pay dividends to shareholders than do right by their employees or the third-world countries they operate in. Luigi explained how, as outlined in the book, banks and corporations don't anticipate these countries paying back their loans. Instead, it's a tactic to secure resources at a cheaper rate. If the leader of the land resists or refuses to comply, they are often replaced or eliminated, with a more compliant figure propped up in their place.

I responded that this made sense, as it explains the stark discrepancies between the "haves" and "have-nots" and why corruption runs rampant in these regions. Ultimately, if leaders don't comply and take the money, they risk being ousted and left with nothing. I admitted that I could see myself being tempted in such circumstances, especially when coming from nothing. How could one not be tempted by such an offer?

We also discussed the dark side of technology. Luigi remarked that while these companies could easily do right by the people in these countries with the profits they make, greed has corrupted their hearts and minds. He said it wouldn't be too much to ensure clean water for the people, to stop polluting rivers with toxic waste, and to provide decent wages all while still making a reasonable profit. Instead, insisted more of humanity is lost with every life impacted or destroyed by these exploitative practices, directly or indirectly.

Luigi's understood and reflected on how societal systems perpetuated inequality. He talked about how he had personally experienced the shortcomings of healthcare, recounting times when he had been overcharged for procedures that seemed routine or necessary. With clear anger in his tone, he once expressed that it wasn't just about him; the system was designed so that only the privileged could survive while the rest of us carried the weight of their greed.

In a WhatsApp voice memo from 2024, Luigi reflected on the consequences of his choices and the lives he had touched. He mentioned that ghosting wasn't really about other people; it was more about creating the space of security in yourself.

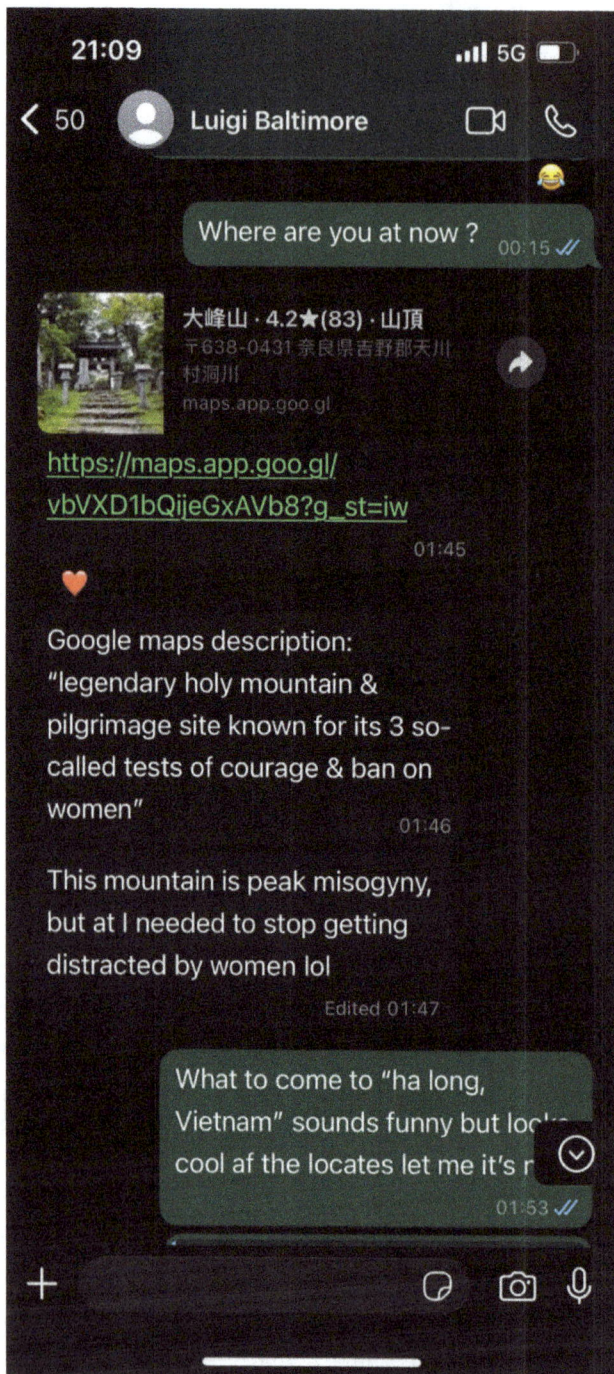

21:09     ..ıll 5G 🔋

‹ 50   👤   **Luigi Baltimore**    🎥   📞

😂

Where are you at now ?   00:15 ✓✓

大峰山 · 4.2★(83) · 山頂
〒638-0431 奈良県吉野郡天川
村洞川
maps.app.goo.gl

https://maps.app.goo.gl/
vbVXD1bQijeGxAVb8?g_st=iw

01:45

❤️

Google maps description:
"legendary holy mountain &
pilgrimage site known for its 3 so-
called tests of courage & ban on
women"

01:46

This mountain is peak misogyny,
but at I needed to stop getting
distracted by women lol

Edited 01:47

What to come to "ha long,
Vietnam" sounds funny but loc[?]
cool af the locates let me it's n[?]

01:53 ✓✓

＋             🏷️   📷   🎤

## Voice Memo: Luigi's Zen Realization

One of the most revealing moments came in a voice memo Luigi sent me in May 2024. He was in Japan at the time, exploring the mountains in Nara. His words captured both his he need for peace and desire find himself:

> *"So, I'm here in the mountains in Nara, and it's fucking beautiful, man. Super lush, like there's this beautiful river that cuts through the gorge, and I've just been like really just zenning out. I think I'm gonna stay here for like—I think I want to stay here for like maybe a month and just like meditate, just hot spring and do some writing. So anyway, we'll go on. So, I realized that today, and I was like, I should reach out about Vietnam. Vietnam sounds like a lot of fun, dude, but yeah, it's like I had a lot of chaos in Thailand—it was great—and now I'm like, I think I want some time to zen out. So, I definitely make it out to Vietnam at some point in the future, but it just doesn't seem like now is, um, that's what I need. So, I'm just gonna zen out and do some, uh, do some Buddha."*
>
> *-Luigi M.*

*Partial quotes in NYTIMES article "Months Before C.E.O.'s Killing, the Suspect Went. Where Was He?"*

We he spoke then he seemed in good spirits and had positive nature about is tone. From my perspective he sounded like he was really getting a much-needed cleanse from technology and time to read, explore, and do hot springs. At the time I did not getting any inclination that he had any issues. He sounded solid; he and I understood the need to be in a high paced area because the temptation to go out into the nightlife can be quite strong because in concreated areas it's hard to except it.

## Luigi's Legacy of Restlessness

The Luigi I knew was complex and had many layers to him. He admired technology but worried about its impact on humanity. He chased freedom but did not mine cutting people off for him to find self-peace. As he drifted further into anonymity, he left behind fragments of himself in every place he visited and every person he met.

I remember stating to him on the phone, *"Be careful in your isolation. I like to 'zen out' as well, but human interaction is necessary."* I shared with him that I had two friends who committed suicide after disconnecting and moving to remote places, leaving everything behind in search of something more. I told him, *"If you ever need anything, please reach out, even if it's just to talk. Let me know because I know how lonely it can get in isolation,"* speaking from my own experience.

A few weeks passed, and while we texted frequently, I was surprised to get a video call from Luigi. That call lasted about 48 minutes, and we talked about many of the topics mentioned in the book. He also wanted to reconnect with a friend. I felt that he hadn't spoken with someone intellectually in a while and wanted to some human interaction after living in the mountains of Japan without the internet.

Luigi and myself had similar personality traits to where neither of us liked to stay still; traveling is in our blood. It was what drove him to explore new places and question societal norms. Even as he disappeared into the mountains of Japan he was just traveling to help focus and find himself.

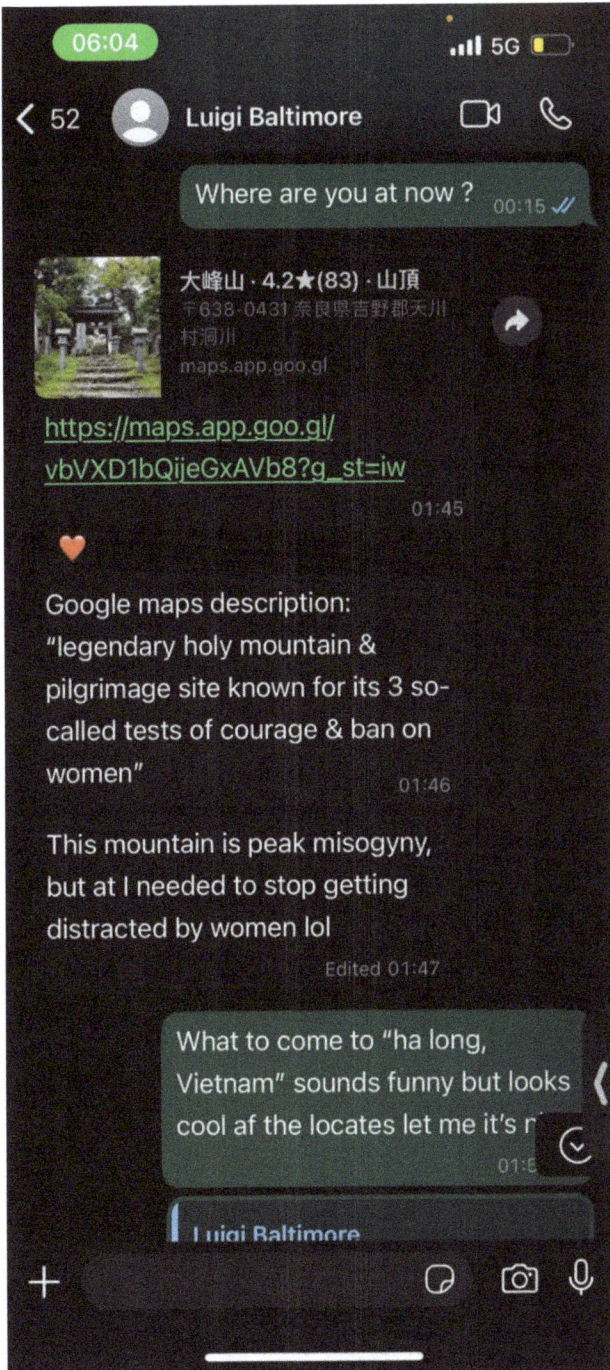

**06:04**    .ıll 5G 🔋

‹ 52   👤  **Luigi Baltimore**    🎥  📞

**Where are you at now ?**  00:15 ✓✓

大峰山 · 4.2★(83) · 山頂
〒638-0431 奈良県吉野郡天川
村洞川
maps.app.goo.gl

https://maps.app.goo.gl/
vbVXD1bQijeGxAVb8?g_st=iw

01:45

❤️

Google maps description:
"legendary holy mountain &
pilgrimage site known for its 3 so-
called tests of courage & ban on
women"    01:46

This mountain is peak misogyny,
but at I needed to stop getting
distracted by women lol

Edited 01:47

What to come to "ha long,
Vietnam" sounds funny but looks
cool af the locates let me it's r
01:5

I Luiai Baltimore

➕                    🏷️  📷  🎤

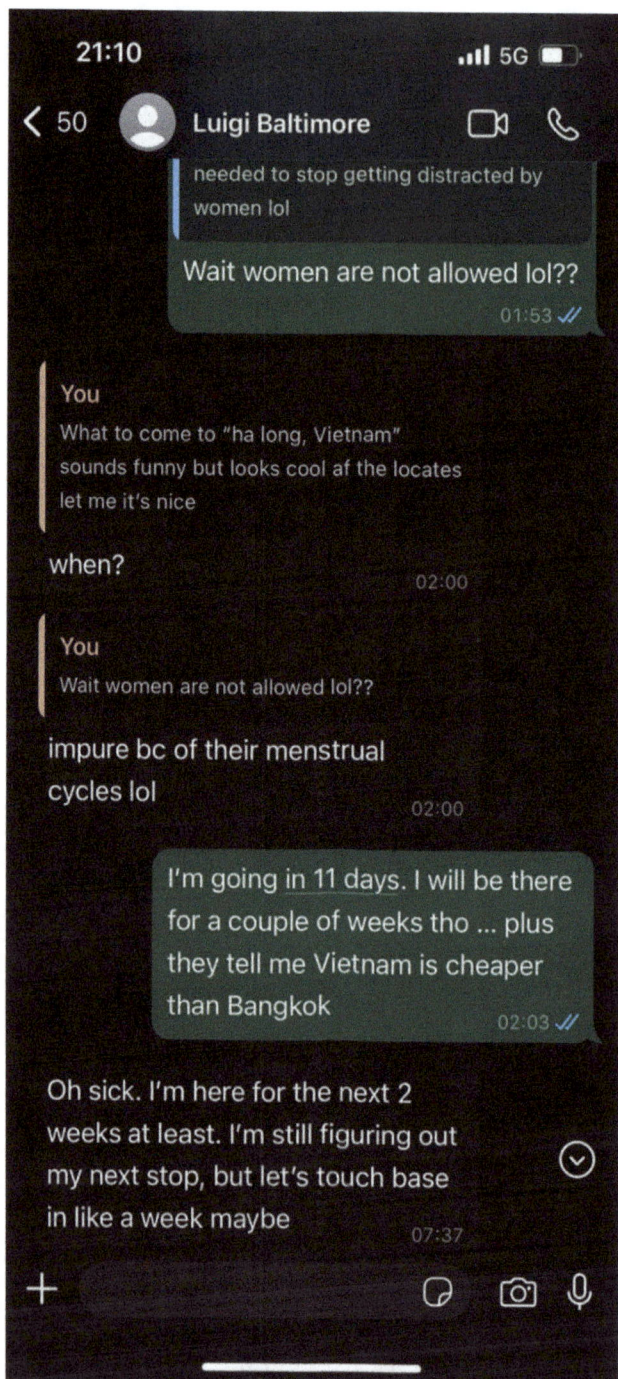

**21:10**  •ııl 5G 🔋

< 50  👤  **Luigi Baltimore**  📹  📞

needed to stop getting distracted by women lol

Wait women are not allowed lol??

01:53 ✓✓

**You**

What to come to "ha long, Vietnam" sounds funny but looks cool af the locates let me it's nice

when?

02:00

**You**

Wait women are not allowed lol??

impure bc of their menstrual cycles lol

02:00

I'm going in 11 days. I will be there for a couple of weeks tho ... plus they tell me Vietnam is cheaper than Bangkok

02:03 ✓✓

Oh sick. I'm here for the next 2 weeks at least. I'm still figuring out my next stop, but let's touch base in like a week maybe

07:37

+  💬  📷  🎤

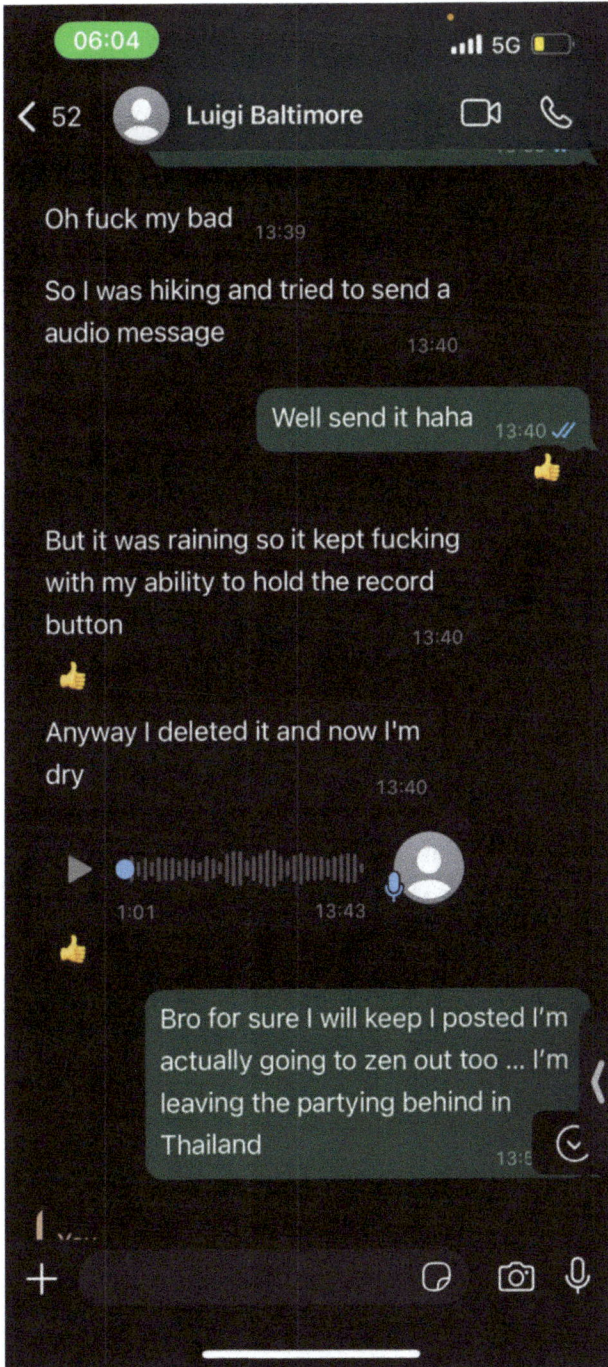

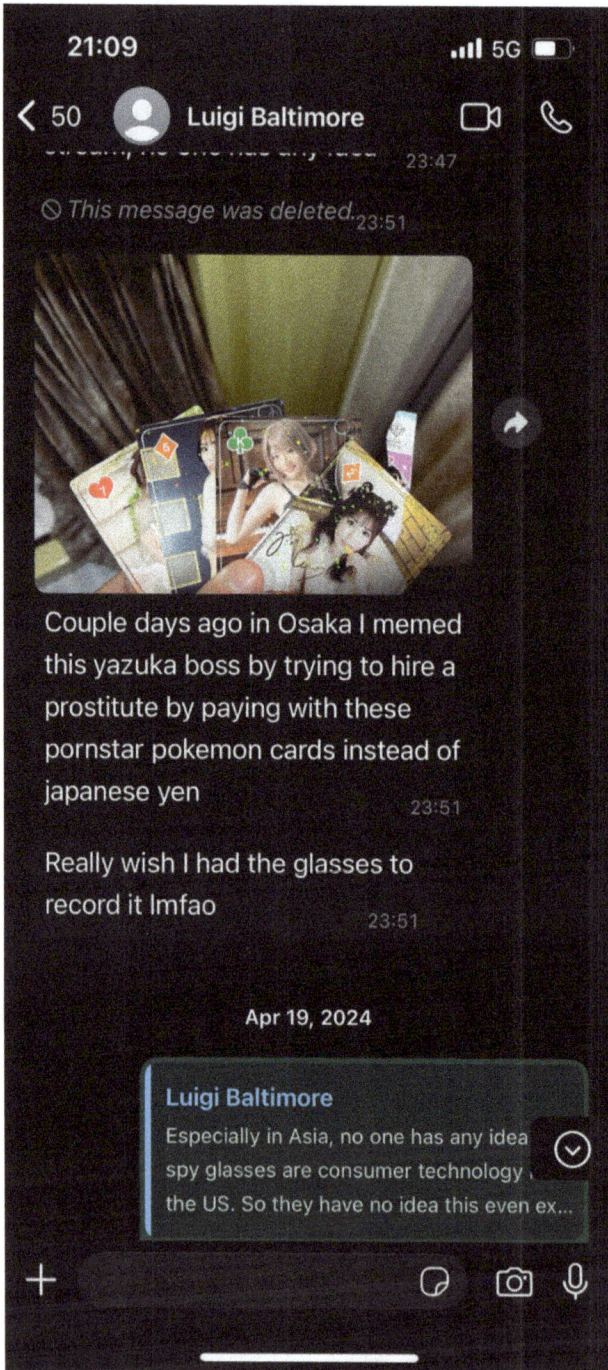

Couple days ago in Osaka I memed this yazuka boss by trying to hire a prostitute by paying with these pornstar pokemon cards instead of japanese yen

23:51

Really wish I had the glasses to record it lmfao

23:51

Apr 19, 2024

**Luigi Baltimore**
Especially in Asia, no one has any idea spy glasses are consumer technology the US. So they have no idea this even ex...

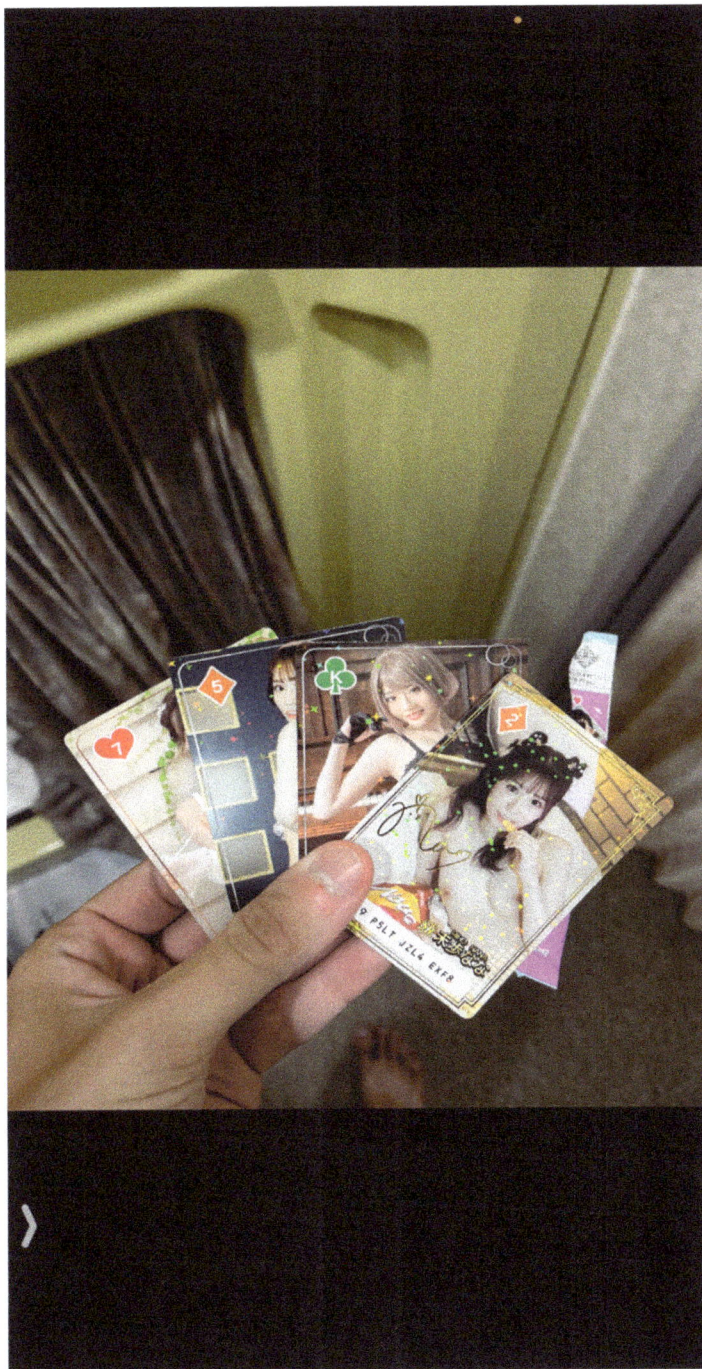

# Chapter 5

# The Final Stretch

By the time Luigi and I had our final conversation, his detachment had deepened. The spoke of plans that were grand in scope but vague in detail. He wanted to travel more, to explore remote corners of the world where he could disconnect from the chaos of modern life. He mentioned that he felt the need to disappear for a while. He wanted to disconnect from phones and deadlines and just have some space to think.

Luigi's distrust of institutions seemed to have intensified. Paraphrasing, he expressed how he saw societal systems healthcare, education, politics as mechanisms designed to keep people chasing things that don't matter. Keeping people locked down in a system and with the invention and the evolution of ai then all human decisions will be created by and algorithm.

Another time, we had a call. He asked me if I really think people can ever change. Or are we all just stuck playing the same roles again and again? His belief as if he wanted to believe in transformation but was unsure.

Luigi's desire for isolation wasn't just a way to escape but rather separate from the noise of modern life, and reconnect with something more primal and authentic. Paraphrasing his thoughts, he often spoke about the beauty of silence, of places untouched by technology and industry. He believed peace wasn't something you found; it was something you created by letting go.

As his plans to withdraw took shape, his presence in our lives became more sporadic as we started speaking less and less. In addition to he being more distance I was a well as in the summer last months I spent in France and Spain.

# Chapter 6

# The Aftermath

When news of Luigi Mangione's alleged involvement in the death of UnitedHealthcare CEO Brian Thompson broke, it felt like the world stopped spinning for a moment. I remember sitting in my apartment in Da Nang, frozen as the headlines flashed across my screen. "How could this be real?" I asked myself over and over again. The man I had known was now the focal point of an international scandal. The world was painting him as a criminal mastermind, but the Luigi I knew was far from that person. He was complex, deeply flawed, and restless but never violent.

As the media frenzy unfolded, I found myself at the center of it, an unintentional link to the man everyone wanted to understand. Within hours of the news breaking, my inbox was flooded with messages from journalists. Andre Tinko from CBS News was the first to reach out, asking if I had known Luigi during his travels. Before I could process his email, others followed. Alondra Valle, ABC News, Good Morning America, Victoria Cox from Insider Edition sent a direct message on Instagram, while Nicholas Bogel-Burroughs from The New York Times contacted me through Instagram. His message was meticulous, detailing his interest in Luigi's personality and mindset during our time in Thailand.

Luigi was one of the smartest people I'd ever met, and for him to get caught at a McDonald's of all places, it just didn't add up. We'd had so many conversations about how processed food was slowly killing people, and he was deeply critical of the food industry. Luigi understood the insidious relationship between the food and healthcare industries and how the former profits from selling unhealthy products while the latter benefits from the resulting health issues. We rarely ate fast food unless one of us had a rare craving, so for him to be there, eating McDonald's seemed completely out of character. It was as if something had snapped, or there was a piece of the story I was missing.

The irony deepened when I learned he was caught with Monopoly money in his possession. It reminded me of the countless times we joked about the currency in Thailand. The colorful bills pink, yellow, and orange felt like play money, especially with the currency conversion rates making everything feel intangible. We often laughed about how spending baht was like playing Monopoly in real life. It was surreal to imagine that something we had joked about so casually had become part of the narrative surrounding his capture.

Even more baffling was how someone as intelligent as Luigi could end up in this situation at all. This was a man who had counseled at Stanford, had an advanced career in AI, and understood the intricate layers of technology and systems better than most people ever could. He was Dr. House-level smart almost too sharp for his own mind at times. Luigi knew how to think through problems and plan meticulously. If he had truly committed a crime, he would have known how to avoid getting caught. We'd all seen shows like *The First 48* and knew the basic rules: get rid of the weapon, don't leave a trail, and disappear. For him to allegedly have the weapon still in his possession was incomprehensible.

The more I think about it, the less sense it makes. Was there a larger game at play? Did something break in his mind? Or am I simply missing a vital piece of the puzzle? Knowing the Luigi I did, none of these fits. It's almost as if the person I knew and the person in the headlines are two entirely different people. The contradictions are too glaring, and even now, I struggle to think of him committing this crime.

Their questions unearthed memories I hadn't revisited in months. As I tried to answer their inquiries, I realized just how much of Luigi's life had remained a mystery to me, even during the time we had spent together. The man I had known in Bangkok was layered, enigmatic, and deeply introspective, but the world now wanted to understand him through the narrow lens of his alleged crime.

Through conversations with these journalists, I learned more about Luigi's movements in the months following our time in Thailand. He had been seen using aliases in Thailand and Japan, blending into the backdrop of each place he visited. The name he shared with me his real name was a rarity. For most people, Luigi met he never spoke to them after the initial connection.

For me, though, Luigi had been more than a passing acquaintance. Our connection felt genuine, even we lost consistency of talking in the later years of the year. The realization that I had been one of the last people Luigi truly opened up to weighed heavily on me. I found myself replaying his voice memos, particularly one he had sent during our time together. You know, man, freedom is a mirage. You chase it and chase it, and when you think you've found it, it disappears. So why not just stop running?

Did Luigi actually commit this crime? It's a question I've wrestled with since the moment his name was tied to the tragedy. Luigi was a mini genius; someone whose intelligence and meticulous nature made it hard to imagine him making a misstep. The very idea that he would commit a crime, let alone leave behind the evidence to implicate himself, feels deeply unsettling. Yet, at the same time, could he be a fall guy? His outspoken views on healthcare his anger at the corruption, greed, and exploitation of people could have made him a target. It's a thought that lingers in the back of my mind.

The healthcare system isn't short on enemies, from frustrated patients to disillusioned doctors. Luigi's stance was far from unique in its criticism, but his clarity and conviction in voicing his disdain stood out. I know doctors who hate working with insurance companies; who doesn't? To be quite honest, I have yet to hear anyone tell me a positive story about an insurance company. Luigi's critiques weren't just general gripes; they were rooted in logic, empathy, and a desire for a system that genuinely cared for people. Could such a bold and unfiltered perspective have made him a scapegoat? It's not impossible.

At the same time, I can't dismiss the reality that there are countless motives among people in the healthcare and insurance industries who might benefit from silencing dissent or shifting blame. Healthcare is a multi-billion-dollar industry, and power doesn't change hands lightly. To think that Luigi's alleged actions were entirely personal feels like ignoring the larger forces at play. The truth is murky, and as much as I want to believe in Luigi's innocence, the weight of the accusations is hard to ignore.

As we watch this case unfold, I hope we can uncover the truth of what really happened. Was Luigi truly the man responsible, or was he caught in a web of circumstances that went far beyond him? Whatever the outcome, the tragedy of it all remains undeniable. A life was lost, and a brilliant mind is now mired in controversy. The system Luigi so passionately criticized has once again taken center stage, and perhaps through this case, we can confront the deeper truths about the broken structures we all live within.

How did we allow this to happen? As citizens, how did we reach a point where someone could feel so overwhelmed by the weight of systemic failures that they might resort to an alleged crime? It's a question that haunts me. It's easy to point fingers, blame the individual, or isolate their actions as a singular event, but the truth is, this is a reflection of something far greater. This is a failure of the systems we've built and sustained.

The cracks in those systems are evident everywhere. We live in a society where healthcare is treated as a privilege, not a right, where people must choose between life-saving treatments and financial ruin, and where the relentless pursuit of profit overshadows the basic tenets of humanity. Insurance companies operate with near impunity, denying claims, raising premiums, and creating a labyrinth of red tape that leaves patients hopelessly entangled. Pharmaceutical companies inflate prices on essential medications, turning what should be accessible treatments into unattainable luxuries for many. Doctors, incentivized by corporate partnerships, are often forced to prioritize what's profitable over what's necessary. Every layer of the system is corrupted, from the top executives to the policies governing it, leaving ordinary people to bear the brunt of the consequences.

And yet, we've allowed it. We've become a society that thrives on distraction, constantly glued to our screens, numbing ourselves with entertainment, sports, and endless social media scrolling. Luigi once remarked how technology has created a kind of mass hypnosis, keeping people so overstimulated that they fail to see the systems operating around them. "If people weren't so consumed by what's on their phones, maybe they'd notice what's happening in the real world," he said. It's a sobering thought, one that forces us to reckon with how much we've let slide while being absorbed in our own lives.

We've let corporations dictate the rules. We've elected leaders who make promises but bend to the will of lobbyists. We've accepted a system that prioritizes shareholders over citizens, one that commodifies health and well-being. How many of us have sat in frustration at a hospital bill, at denied claims, at overpriced prescriptions, and thought, "This can't be right," but then moved on because we felt powerless to change it? That feeling of helplessness is the foundation of a broken system. It thrives because we believe we can't dismantle it.

Luigi understood this deeply. He often spoke about how society has normalized suffering under the guise of progress. Paraphrasing his thoughts, he'd question how we could call ourselves the best system in the world when the system itself seemed designed to harm its people. Luigi would often contrast this with countries where healthcare was accessible and affordable, highlighting the stark disparities.

The pressure of this reality isn't just financial but it's also emotional, psychological, and moral. It weighs on people in ways that are hard to articulate. Imagine knowing that your loved one's life could have been saved but wasn't because of a denied claim or a medication priced out of reach. Imagine seeing the system fail over and over again and feeling like there's no way to fix it. The frustration builds, the anger festers, and for some, the weight becomes unbearable.

How has it come to this? Perhaps it's because we've allowed greed to run unchecked. We've let the pursuit of profit become the ultimate goal, valuing it over human life. We've allowed our political systems to be influenced by corporate interests, silencing the voices of the people in favor of those with the deepest pockets. We've created a world were doing the right thing often feels impossible because the stakes are so high, and the powers that be seem untouchable.

But if we're honest, this isn't just a failure of systems but us as a collective people to allow this problem to persist. It's a failure to hold those in power accountable, a failure to demand better, a failure to recognize our collective responsibility. We've allowed the distractions of modern life to keep us passive, to make us believe that change is beyond our reach. And in doing so, we've allowed the weight of these systems to crush those who can't bear it anymore.

Luigi's story and the tragic circumstances surrounding it are a wake-up call. They force us to confront not just the flaws in our systems but the complacency within ourselves. If we want to prevent more tragedies, more lives lost, and more people pushed to their breaking points, we have to start asking hard questions. How much longer can we let this continue? How many more lives must be affected before we decide that enough is enough? The answers won't come easily, but one thing is clear: the path we're on is unsustainable, and unless we change course, the consequences will only grow more devastating.

# Conclusion: Understanding Luigi

Luigi Mangione was a man who defied easy categorization. He was both open and guarded, restless and reflective, searching for meaning while simultaneously running from it. Writing this book has been my way of reconciling the man I knew with the actions he is accused of. It's not about absolving him or excusing his choices but rather diving into his understanding.

Luigi was not a saint, nor was he a monster. He was human, shaped by a world he often felt at odds with. He was a friend, a thinker, and a rebel, someone who lived on the edges of society, questioning its structures and seeking truths.

As I reflect on our time together, I'm left with more questions than answers. But perhaps that's fitting. Luigi was never one to be easily understood, and maybe that's what made him so unforgettable. His story, like all our stories, is a tapestry of experiences, choices, and emotions a reminder that even the most extraordinary lives are still deeply human.

This book is not just about Luigi; it's about the systems, circumstances, and choices that shape us all. It's a story of freedom and constraint, of searching and fleeing, of joy and despair. And while Luigi's path ended in tragedy, his journey reminds us of the complexity of the human spirit.

# Self-Reflection

The question that I pose here is: What would push someone to commit alleged murder? I believe everyone knows someone going through health issues where the healthcare system has failed them. Whenever you need surgery and insurance says it's cosmetic, when you need medication but it's not in your tier plan, or when you need surgery, but they give you a budget that's much lower than what the actual surgery costs, or they cap it—these are all ways the system betrays its people. As a nation, we have to do better, especially when we claim to be the greatest.

What we need to do as a nation is self-reflect, look at the need for change, and actually make those changes. There are so many industries that benefit off the backs of people, with corporations placing profit over health, safety, and the environment. Making money is great—it's the American way—but this could be the time we pivot before anyone else loses their life.

I believe America can change, but it will take some brave CEO or executive to stand up and tell the shareholders, "Hey, we're not going for profits, and we're going to be a little less profitable this year because we must invest in areas for our employees and the general public." It would take brave board members to stand by that CEO and not fire or dismiss them in favor of another pro-profit leader. It would take brave groups of politicians on both sides to band together and stand up to corporations that have funded their campaigns—and will fund their opponents' campaigns if their views and policies don't align with corporate goals.

It would take holding people accountable and standing together to ensure these corporations are held responsible for their actions or inactions. It would take whistleblowers who risk their lives to expose the truth about industries that prioritize profit over human well-being.

The tragedy of this is that one must go to such extremes just to do right by people. As a proud American, I enjoy money like the next man, but when will we self-assess and say enough is enough? People mean more than money. We are so advanced as a nation that somewhere along the way, we've forgotten that we are all fellow Americans. I want us to live in a world where an alleged murder does not have to occur because people are feeling frustrated about the system. I want a world where America is not just the greatest at money but the greatest at treating humans like humans. We have the resources. It's not too late for us to change course. Lives are lost every day that benefit others across many industries. Luigi's alleged crime awakened us to something bigger—that we have to have morals over money. When will we prioritize life, health, and safety over the dollar? These are the questions we need to ask ourselves before it's too late.

In the end, this story is not about absolution or condemnation. It's about reflection, understanding, and the urgent need to change the systems that shape our lives. Let this be a call to action for us all to seek compassion, accountability, and a future where tragedies like these no longer have to exist.

# Final Reflections

As I think back on my time with Luigi, I'm struck by his complexity. He was a man of contradictions but one who still believed in hope, a critic who sought solutions, and a wanderer who longed for home. His insights challenged me, his humor disarmed me, and his friendship reminded me of the importance of staying true to oneself. In a world that often feels overwhelming and unjust, Luigi's search for meaning stands as a testament to the resilience of the human spirit. I will watch this trial closely as we can all watch what unfolds.

www.ingramcontent.com/pod-product-compliance
Lightning Source LLC
Chambersburg PA
CBHW070031030426
42335CB00017B/2380